Reversing Chilbl
Filtratio

The Raw Vegan Plant-Based Detoxification & Regeneration Workbook for Healing Patients.

Volume 5

Health Central

This book, with the opinions, suggestions and references made within it, is based on the author's personal experience and is for personal study and research purposes only. This program is about health and vitality, not disease. The author makes no medical claims. If you choose to use the material in this book on yourself, the author and publisher take no responsibility for your actions and decisions or the consequences thereof..

The Importance of Kidneys

Once upon a time, "disease" or dis-ease within the human body did not exist.

Humans lived and passed naturally. It was their ability to live long and healthy lives that allowed for the human race to continue to replicate and evolve. Today we are seeing a different reality unfold.

Our health has become imbalanced because we are no longer consuming the foods intended for us. We are seeing the human body struggle with removing the toxins resulting from this imbalance. This is leading to dysfunction within different locations of the body. Diagnosis of a "disease" follows shortly after.

The location of the dysfunction / dis-ease within your body, whether that is within an organ, gland or nerve, will always stem from the kidneys (and adrenal glands). The key to realise here is that it was a kidney issue before it became a formally labelled "disease".

The kidneys (including the skin) are the main sites where your lymphatic system eliminates its waste and acids. This lymphatic system is your body's sewage system and therefore is responsible for the cleansing of all accumulating waste from tissue and blood.

So when the filtration ability of your kidneys grounds to a halt, your lymphatic system's waste starts to back up and become congested in pockets - this eventually spreads. You now have acids settling into interstitial spaces (in and around the cells) within the tissue.

Any genetic weaknesses that you have inherited will be the first to worsen and develop dis-ease. Extreme environmental factors, such as a mobile phone mast right outside your home – or high levels of hazardous airborne substances, can all play a role in triggering a weakness within your body.

In general, we find that the genetically weak tissue that was inherited tends to be the first to be affected before the issue spreads.

Why?

Now that we understand the role of your kidneys and the importance of them filtering well – we move onto the question of why would your kidneys become impaired?

The human body is formed predominantly of liquid. Therefore retaining a healthy level of hydration is an important consideration. Based on your consumption, you will alter the chemistry within your body. This will either create a positive environment (hydration) or a negative environment (dehydration).

Your inner chemistry consists of two states – Acidic (pH less than 7) or Basic (Alkaline – pH more than 7). We already acknowledge that acids are damaging and dehydrating - they create a cationic (acidic & congested imbalance) environment within you.

The majority of humans today have strayed away from the raw diet intended for us – with most consuming foods that are resulting in the formation of an acidic chemistry. This applies not only to the food and drink that you consume but also anything that you apply to your skin (creams, lotions, soaps, cosmetics) as this is also ingested.

How?

For your tissue and cells to detoxify, heal and regenerate, you must start to drain your lymphatic system through your kidneys. This can only be made possible through a change in diet and daily routine.

We must therefore eliminate all low energy, acid and mucus forming foods from our diets (beans, all animal products: meat, dairy, eggs, all processed/frozen foods, wheat/grains: bread, pasta).

Proteins tend to be very straining on the kidneys. Resultantly your body is infiltrated by uric acid and these acids cause the breakdown of your kidneys whilst mucus and stones are formed.

All of this congestion within the kidneys then causes a significant blockage to the flow of energy through them. Their ability to filter out metabolic waste and toxins is then hindered.

The solution for opening up the kidneys lies with a 100% raw fruit diet, with the occasional vegetables where needed (juiced carrots being extremely healing and regenerative – juiced celery is also powerful).

Herbs

In order to support your kidneys, there are a variety of herbs that can be taken, some of which include: Saw Palmetto, Cleavers, Stinging Nettle, Uva Ursi, Marshmallow Root, Parsley, Dandelion Root, Couch Grass, Corn Silk, Horsetail, Juniper Berries, Goldenrod, Cordyceps.

It should be noted that the adrenal glands and kidneys are very closely related. The adrenal glands sit above the kidneys and produce neurotransmitters that support the activation of kidney filtration. Equally if the kidneys slow down, so do the adrenal glands - they work synergistically (hand-in-hand).

In some cases patients have very weak adrenal glands and this leads to an impaired kidney function. Factors that can cause weakened adrenal glands include: prolonged stress, toxic environments, and a weak pituitary gland.

Some herbs that you could use in order to support adrenal gland health include: Kelp, Ashwagandha, Siberian Ginseng, Ho Shou Wu Root, Liquorice Root, Wild Yam Root, Rhodiola.

Fruits offer high astringent (suction on cells/tissue) and hydration value, and they are the most easily digestible foods, with all nutrients being available for fast absorption (providing that the related organs have been cleansed and are functioning as they should be). We have found grapes and all citrus fruits to be highly astringent and cleansing.

Our earliest ancestors lived off the land and as with all other species, ate a fully raw diet (predominantly fruit with some vegetables) – therefore making them frugivores. All other species retained their species-specific diet whilst the humans ventured off down the road of cooked and processed foods.

When you return to the diet designed just for you and your species, you will feel your body normalise (hydrate) and balance out (alkalise) as your kidneys re-awaken and rid your body of all the accumulated acids. Your colon will also naturally flush itself out.

Real hydration comes through raw living water-dense foods. Cooking out foods destroys this living element and significantly reduces the energy load that the food will provide you – all whilst becoming more energy consuming for your digestive system to process. This is why you feel fatigued after eating a cooked meal.

Timescales

With your organs (including your adrenal glands and kidneys) having been over-worked and weakened – they will not be functioning as they should be. Your lymphatic system will likely be backed up and in some cases stagnant – and your bowels will also be impeded with mucus, mucoid plaque, biofilms (bacteria, fungi), and parasites plastered on their walls.

Therefore, a key concept to understand is that although you will start to feel a difference relatively quickly – you should be prepared for the longer haul in order to witness the more lasting changes within yourself.

The speed of achieving results can be accelerated with intermittent dry fasting (for 16+ hours) and slow juicing fruit (conserves digestive energy) but equally it should be noted that nothing happens over night – especially when you are healing and reversing years of acidity, dehydration and tissue damage. It is important to manage your own expectations here.

Everybody reaches their destination in the end – however long it takes.

The management and conservation of energy within your body is a major contributor of healing. Eating and digesting solid fruit/vegetable matter uses energy, and this energy could be better used re-directed towards healing and regeneration.

So for extreme cases, we prescribe intermittent dry fasting for at least 16 hours (always work your way up) – opened with fruit juice that has been made by using a cold press slow juicer. This is a higher level of detoxification, and with juice, you will experience far more effective nutrient delivery.

Adjust the amount of juice you consume based on how you feel – always listen to your body. It is easy for practitioners to recommend drinking 3 to 5 litres of juice to all patients but in reality, everybody is different and there are too many factors involved to make such a generalised recommendation. Factors such as: age, height, weight, body fat percentage, body type, current organ weaknesses.

If you are not in a critical state, it would be better for you to slowly transition into a fruit diet. Once you are fully fruit, maintain this routine for a month or two before introducing intermittent dry fasting which will really help to further open up your kidneys and drain out the acidic waste from your body.

The skin (known as the 3rd kidney) can also drain your lymphatic system's waste through deep sweat (sauna or a hot climate) – contributing to the fight against systemic acidosis.

Open up all of your kidneys and filtration channels - and you will soon witness the positive changes that you desire.

Good luck – stay focused – remain persistent - it's very simple and easy.

Wishing you all the best and if you would like to book a consultation or have any queries, thoughts, feedback / comments, feel free to email us at:

HealingCentral8@gmail.com

Good Luck with your healing journey.

The Power of Journaling

Journaling your inner self talk is a truly effective way of increasing self awareness and consciousness. To be able to transfer your thoughts and feelings onto a piece of paper is a really effective method of self reflection and improvement. This is much needed when you are switching to a high fruit dietary routine.

You are welcome to add notes on any spaces you find within this book – or alternatively you can use a basic notepad. Be sure to add the date of journaling at the top of each page used. This is invaluable for when you wish to go back and review your feelings and thoughts on previous dates.

Keep a comprehensive record of activities, thoughts, and really log everything you ate/are eating. You can even make miscellaneous notes if you feel that they will help you.

I like to use journals to have a conversation with myself. Inner talk can really help you overcome any challenges that you are experiencing. Express yourself and any concerns that you may have.

Try to advise yourself as though you are your best friend – similarly to how you would advise a close friend or family member. You will be surprised at the results that you will achieve from using this technique.

We have laid out the following examples of different ways that you could complete your daily journaling with the support of this book. These are just basic examples – you can complete your daily journals in any other way that you feel is most comfortable for you.

[EXAMPLE 1]

Today's Date: 6th May 2018

Morning

I just ate 3 mangoes - very sweet and tasty. I felt a heavy feeling under my chest area so I stopped eating. Unsure what that was - maybe digestive or the transverse colon?

Afternoon

I was feeling hungry so I am eating some dried figs, pineapple and apricots with around 750ml of spring water.

Evening

Sipping on a green tea (herbal). Feeling pretty strong and alert at the moment.

Night

Enjoying a bowl of red seeded grapes. Currently I feel satisfied.

Today's Notes (Highlights, Thoughts, Feelings):

Unlike yesterday, today was a good day. I am noticing an increase in regular bowel movements which makes me feel cleansed and light afterwards. I feel as though my kidneys are also starting to filter better (white sediment visible in morning wee).

It definitely helps to document my thoughts in this workbook. A great way to reflect, improve and stay on track.

Feeling very good - vibrant and strong - I have noticed a major improvement in my physical fitness and performance. Mentally I feel healthier and happier.

[EXAMPLE 2]

Today's Date: 7th May 2018

Morning

Dry fasting (water and food free since 8pm last night) - will go up until 12:30pm today, and start with 500ml of spring water before eating half a watermelon.

Afternoon

Kept busy and was in and out quite a bit – so nothing consumed.

Evening

At around 5pm, I had a peppermint tea with a selection of mixed dried fruit (small bowl of apricot, dates, mango, pineapple, and prunes).

Night

Sipped on spring water through the evening as required.
Finished off the other half of the watermelon from the morning.

Today's Notes (Highlights, Thoughts, Feelings):

As with most days, today started well with me dry fasting (continuing my fast from my sleep/skipping breakfast) up until around 12:30pm and then eating half a watermelon. The laxative effect of the watermelon helped me poop and release any loosened toxins from the fasting period.
I tend to struggle on some days from 3pm onwards. Up until that point I am okay but if the cravings strike then it can be challenging. I remind myself that those burgers and chips do not have any live healing energy.
I feel good in general. I feel fantastic doing a fruit/juice fast but slightly empty by the end of the day.
Cooked food makes me feel severe fatigue and mental fog.
Will continue with my fruit fasting and start to introduce fruit juices due to their deeper detox benefits. I would love to be on juices only as I have seen others within the community achieve amazing results.

[EXAMPLE 3]

Today's Date: 8th May 2018

Morning

Today I woke and my children were enjoying some watermelon for breakfast – and the smell was luring so I joined them. Large bowl of watermelon eaten at around 8am. Started with a glass of water.

Afternoon

Snacked on left over watermelon throughout the morning and afternoon. Had 5 dates an hour or so after.

Evening

Had around 3 mangoes at around 6pm. Felt content – but then I was invited round to a family gathering where a selection of pizzas, burgers and chips were being served. I gave into the peer pressure and felt like I let myself down!

Night

Having over-eaten earlier on in the evening, I was still feeling bloated with a headache (possibly digestion related) and I also felt quite mucus filled (wheez in chest and coughing up phlegm). Very sleepy and low energy. The perils of cooked foods!!

Today's Notes (Highlights, Thoughts, Feelings):

I let myself down today. It all started well until I ate a fully blown meal (and over-ate). I didn't remain focussed and I spun off track. As a result my energy levels were much lower and I felt a bout of extreme fatigue 30 minutes after the meal (most likely the body struggling to with digesting all that cooked food).
I need to stick to the plan because the difference between fruit fasting, and eating cooked foods is huge – 1 makes you feel empowered whilst the other makes you feel drained. I also felt the mucus overload after the meal – it kicked in pretty quickly.
Today I felt disappointed after giving in to the meal but tomorrow is a new day and I will keep on going! It is important to remind myself that I won't get better if I cannot stick to the routine.

Frequently Asked Questions

1. Will this really work for me?
Yes. We are sent this question quite often. The reason why the prospect of eating a high fruit raw diet is so daunting and strange to us is because we have been so heavily brainwashed by the norms of society. Advertising of the latest food trends has hypnotised us and so we are no longer able to see through our self-formed reality. Our family's eating trends also play a role in our belief that we must eat in a certain way. Social eating is another major contributor to this. Eating raw fruit and vegetables from the land is the diet intended for our species. As children, we were naturally attracted towards fruit over cooked foods. However, the only way to develop belief in this way of eating is to experience it first-hand – try eating a fruit-only diet of your favourite fruit for 3 days, and take a note of; how you feel, your sleep quality, your energy levels, digestion and elimination – give it a go, you have nothing to lose, and everything to gain. You will naturally come to the conclusion that it works for you.

2. Will your other book volumes help me?
Yes. We have covered a variety of unique topics in the different book volumes found in this series. Each is geared around educating and supporting you in reaching your goals of good health and being "disease" free. Going from years of eating a mucus-forming diet - to eating fully raw - you should be informed about the different aspects of this any new protocol. There are many areas and angles within the scope of normalising your body's state and ridding it of "disease". You will also find different Frequently Asked Questions (sent in to us by readers) in each book and these question-and-answer sections are very insightful and helpful. In summary, the different book volumes will guide and support you through your healing journey.

3. My MD (Medical Doctor) is encouraging me to stick to my current diet and medication schedule. What should I do?
This is a very good question as it is a common topic that we face on a daily basis. We do not advise you to stop taking your medicines. We suggest that you change your diet and assure your MD that you will continue to take the prescribed medicines in your new dietary routine. Also ask to have a review of your medicines every 3 to 4 weeks because as your health improves and you strengthen, you will inevitably need less medication. You can discuss the reduction of medicines with your MD at these appointments. Keep in mind that MDs are not trained on nutrition and cure – but more so on medicines and symptom suppression/management. Cure yourself and become the example for your MD to learn from.
For fruit juicing: **YourFruitJuicer.com**
For vegetable juicing: **YourVegJuicer.com**

DAY STRUCTURE REMINDERS

For The Morning...

Continuing your dry fast from your night sleep is a good idea. Work towards fasting up until at least 12pm. As your body adapts, start to increase this - the later you break your fast - the better.

In The Afternoon...

When you do finally decide to open your fast - focus on hydration. Spring water is a good start or slow-juiced fruits (e.g. berries, melons, citrus). Alternatively, eating soaked dates or your favourite fruits will suffice.

Evening Feast...

Work towards dry fasting for 23 hours and eating for 1 hour each day. This will take time to reach - listen to your body and get there in your own pace. The ideal time to break your dry fast would be approximately 6pm to 7pm

And At Night Time...

Be sure to completely stop eating by 8pm (latest) so your body can prepare for a good night's sleep, rest and recovery.

DAY 1: DAILY TIP

"Take a herbal parasite formula for at least a month whilst on a fruit-only diet. It will help with eliminating food cravings and desires for specific "junk" foods. Eradicating parasites will significantly ease your journey"

DAY STRUCTURE REMINDERS

For The Morning...

Continuing your dry fast from your night sleep is a good idea. Work towards fasting up until at least 12pm. As your body adapts, start to increase this - the later you break your fast - the better.

In The Afternoon...

When you do finally decide to open your fast - focus on hydration. Spring water is a good start or slow-juiced fruits (e.g. berries, melons, citrus). Alternatively, eating soaked dates or your favourite fruits will suffice.

Evening Feast...

Work towards dry fasting for 23 hours and eating for 1 hour each day. This will take time to reach - listen to your body and get there in your own pace. The ideal time to break your dry fast would be approximately 6pm to 7pm

And At Night Time...

Be sure to completely stop eating by 8pm (latest) so your body can prepare for a good night's sleep, rest and recovery.

DAY 2: DAILY TIP

"Your skin is the largest eliminative organ that you possess. Skin brushing and sweating are crucial to support the detoxification phase. Sauna heat or a hot climate work well. A steam room can also help if the others are not available."

DAY STRUCTURE REMINDERS

For The Morning...

Continuing your dry fast from your night sleep is a good idea. Work towards fasting up until at least 12pm. As your body adapts, start to increase this - the later you break your fast - the better.

In The Afternoon...

When you do finally decide to open your fast - focus on hydration. Spring water is a good start or slow-juiced fruits (e.g. berries, melons, citrus). Alternatively, eating soaked dates or your favourite fruits will suffice.

Evening Feast...

Work towards dry fasting for 23 hours and eating for 1 hour each day. This will take time to reach - listen to your body and get there in your own pace. The ideal time to break your dry fast would be approximately 6pm to 7pm

And At Night Time...

Be sure to completely stop eating by 8pm (latest) so your body can prepare for a good night's sleep, rest and recovery.

DAY 3: DAILY TIP

"If you are on medications, closely monitor the relevant statistics (e.g. blood pressure, blood sugar level, etc) on a regular basis. Have blood tests carried out where necessary. Upon improving, reduce your medication accordingly"

DAY STRUCTURE REMINDERS

For The Morning...

Continuing your dry fast from your night sleep is a good idea. Work towards fasting up until at least 12pm. As your body adapts, start to increase this - the later you break your fast - the better.

In The Afternoon...

When you do finally decide to open your fast - focus on hydration. Spring water is a good start or slow-juiced fruits (e.g. berries, melons, citrus). Alternatively, eating soaked dates or your favourite fruits will suffice.

Evening Feast...

Work towards dry fasting for 23 hours and eating for 1 hour each day. This will take time to reach - listen to your body and get there in your own pace. The ideal time to break your dry fast would be approximately 6pm to 7pm

And At Night Time...

Be sure to completely stop eating by 8pm (latest) so your body can prepare for a good night's sleep, rest and recovery.

DAY 4: DAILY TIP

"Most people do not breathe effectively. Your body requires a healthy supply of oxygen in order to heal. Practice breathing (5 seconds in/5 seconds out) daily. If it is possible, perform deep breathing exercises by the sea or green nature."

DAY STRUCTURE REMINDERS

For The Morning...

Continuing your dry fast from your night sleep is a good idea. Work towards fasting up until at least 12pm. As your body adapts, start to increase this - the later you break your fast - the better.

In The Afternoon...

When you do finally decide to open your fast - focus on hydration. Spring water is a good start or slow-juiced fruits (e.g. berries, melons, citrus). Alternatively, eating soaked dates or your favourite fruits will suffice.

Evening Feast...

Work towards dry fasting for 23 hours and eating for 1 hour each day. This will take time to reach - listen to your body and get there in your own pace. The ideal time to break your dry fast would be approximately 6pm to 7pm

And At Night Time...

Be sure to completely stop eating by 8pm (latest) so your body can prepare for a good night's sleep, rest and recovery.

DAY 5: DAILY TIP

"Disease is not the presence of something evil, but rather the lack of the presence of something essential."

— Dr. Bernard Jensen.

DAY STRUCTURE REMINDERS

For The Morning...

Continuing your dry fast from your night sleep is a good idea. Work towards fasting up until at least 12pm. As your body adapts, start to increase this - the later you break your fast - the better.

In The Afternoon...

When you do finally decide to open your fast - focus on hydration. Spring water is a good start or slow-juiced fruits (e.g. berries, melons, citrus). Alternatively, eating soaked dates or your favourite fruits will suffice.

Evening Feast...

Work towards dry fasting for 23 hours and eating for 1 hour each day. This will take time to reach - listen to your body and get there in your own pace. The ideal time to break your dry fast would be approximately 6pm to 7pm

And At Night Time...

Be sure to completely stop eating by 8pm (latest) so your body can prepare for a good night's sleep, rest and recovery.

DAY 6: DAILY TIP

"Fruits are empowering. They will energise you with live electrical energy. Cooked foods in comparison will use your vital energy stores on digestion - leaving you feeling fatigued. We want this energy reserved for healing."

DAY STRUCTURE REMINDERS

For The Morning...

Continuing your dry fast from your night sleep is a good idea. Work towards fasting up until at least 12pm. As your body adapts, start to increase this - the later you break your fast - the better.

In The Afternoon...

When you do finally decide to open your fast - focus on hydration. Spring water is a good start or slow-juiced fruits (e.g. berries, melons, citrus). Alternatively, eating soaked dates or your favourite fruits will suffice.

Evening Feast...

Work towards dry fasting for 23 hours and eating for 1 hour each day. This will take time to reach - listen to your body and get there in your own pace. The ideal time to break your dry fast would be approximately 6pm to 7pm

And At Night Time...

Be sure to completely stop eating by 8pm (latest) so your body can prepare for a good night's sleep, rest and recovery.

DAY 7: DAILY TIP

"Fructose (the sugar found in fruits) is kind to the pancreas and its absorption into the cells/body uses minimal energy. It is also extremely cleansing for the gut."

DAY STRUCTURE REMINDERS

For The Morning...

Continuing your dry fast from your night sleep is a good idea. Work towards fasting up until at least 12pm. As your body adapts, start to increase this - the later you break your fast - the better.

In The Afternoon...

When you do finally decide to open your fast - focus on hydration. Spring water is a good start or slow-juiced fruits (e.g. berries, melons, citrus). Alternatively, eating soaked dates or your favourite fruits will suffice.

Evening Feast...

Work towards dry fasting for 23 hours and eating for 1 hour each day. This will take time to reach - listen to your body and get there in your own pace. The ideal time to break your dry fast would be approximately 6pm to 7pm

And At Night Time...

Be sure to completely stop eating by 8pm (latest) so your body can prepare for a good night's sleep, rest and recovery.

DAY 8: DAILY TIP

"Fruits have the highest healing energy frequencies among all food groups. Vegetables are the next highest. Cooked meats rank the lowest."

DAY STRUCTURE REMINDERS

For The Morning...

Continuing your dry fast from your night sleep is a good idea. Work towards fasting up until at least 12pm. As your body adapts, start to increase this - the later you break your fast - the better.

In The Afternoon...

When you do finally decide to open your fast - focus on hydration. Spring water is a good start or slow-juiced fruits (e.g. berries, melons, citrus). Alternatively, eating soaked dates or your favourite fruits will suffice.

Evening Feast...

Work towards dry fasting for 23 hours and eating for 1 hour each day. This will take time to reach - listen to your body and get there in your own pace. The ideal time to break your dry fast would be approximately 6pm to 7pm

And At Night Time...

Be sure to completely stop eating by 8pm (latest) so your body can prepare for a good night's sleep, rest and recovery.

DAY 9: DAILY TIP

"Mucus congestion (caused by animal and wheat based products) leads to a lack of mineral utilization (Calcium, Magnesium, Potassium, etc). This leads to weakened bones and teeth amongst other weaknesses."

DAY STRUCTURE REMINDERS

For The Morning...

Continuing your dry fast from your night sleep is a good idea. Work towards fasting up until at least 12pm. As your body adapts, start to increase this - the later you break your fast - the better.

In The Afternoon...

When you do finally decide to open your fast - focus on hydration. Spring water is a good start or slow-juiced fruits (e.g. berries, melons, citrus). Alternatively, eating soaked dates or your favourite fruits will suffice.

Evening Feast...

Work towards dry fasting for 23 hours and eating for 1 hour each day. This will take time to reach - listen to your body and get there in your own pace. The ideal time to break your dry fast would be approximately 6pm to 7pm

And At Night Time...

Be sure to completely stop eating by 8pm (latest) so your body can prepare for a good night's sleep, rest and recovery.

DAY 10: DAILY TIP

"Did you know that the juice of oranges, and kale (slow juiced) will offer you more biologically available Calcium than Cow's Milk? There will also be no mucus or acid formation with this fruit / vegetable juice."

DAY STRUCTURE REMINDERS

For The Morning...

Continuing your dry fast from your night sleep is a good idea. Work towards fasting up until at least 12pm. As your body adapts, start to increase this - the later you break your fast - the better.

In The Afternoon...

When you do finally decide to open your fast - focus on hydration. Spring water is a good start or slow-juiced fruits (e.g. berries, melons, citrus). Alternatively, eating soaked dates or your favourite fruits will suffice.

Evening Feast...

Work towards dry fasting for 23 hours and eating for 1 hour each day. This will take time to reach - listen to your body and get there in your own pace. The ideal time to break your dry fast would be approximately 6pm to 7pm

And At Night Time...

Be sure to completely stop eating by 8pm (latest) so your body can prepare for a good night's sleep, rest and recovery.

DAY 11: DAILY TIP

"Your body will use sweating (fevers), vomiting, diarrhea, frequent urination, colds, flus, and regular bowel movements as a means to detoxify your acidic state. Do not be alarmed - let it run its course."

DAY STRUCTURE REMINDERS

For The Morning...

Continuing your dry fast from your night sleep is a good idea. Work towards fasting up until at least 12pm. As your body adapts, start to increase this - the later you break your fast - the better.

In The Afternoon...

When you do finally decide to open your fast - focus on hydration. Spring water is a good start or slow-juiced fruits (e.g. berries, melons, citrus). Alternatively, eating soaked dates or your favourite fruits will suffice.

Evening Feast...

Work towards dry fasting for 23 hours and eating for 1 hour each day. This will take time to reach - listen to your body and get there in your own pace. The ideal time to break your dry fast would be approximately 6pm to 7pm

And At Night Time...

Be sure to completely stop eating by 8pm (latest) so your body can prepare for a good night's sleep, rest and recovery.

DAY 12: DAILY TIP

"Pain is merely a sign of energy blockage(s) resulting from acidosis. Alkalization and hydration hold the key (through detoxification) for the removal of dysfunction and imbalances to take place."

DAY STRUCTURE REMINDERS

For The Morning...

Continuing your dry fast from your night sleep is a good idea. Work towards fasting up until at least 12pm. As your body adapts, start to increase this - the later you break your fast - the better.

In The Afternoon...

When you do finally decide to open your fast - focus on hydration. Spring water is a good start or slow-juiced fruits (e.g. berries, melons, citrus). Alternatively, eating soaked dates or your favourite fruits will suffice.

Evening Feast...

Work towards dry fasting for 23 hours and eating for 1 hour each day. This will take time to reach - listen to your body and get there in your own pace. The ideal time to break your dry fast would be approximately 6pm to 7pm

And At Night Time...

Be sure to completely stop eating by 8pm (latest) so your body can prepare for a good night's sleep, rest and recovery.

DAY 13: DAILY TIP

"Keep on loving! Love is alkalizing, it improves digestion and kidney elimination. Your blood and lymph flow will also improve as a result. Start to love and care selflessly and reap the rewards."

DAY STRUCTURE REMINDERS

For The Morning...

Continuing your dry fast from your night sleep is a good idea. Work towards fasting up until at least 12pm. As your body adapts, start to increase this - the later you break your fast - the better.

In The Afternoon...

When you do finally decide to open your fast - focus on hydration. Spring water is a good start or slow-juiced fruits (e.g. berries, melons, citrus). Alternatively, eating soaked dates or your favourite fruits will suffice.

Evening Feast...

Work towards dry fasting for 23 hours and eating for 1 hour each day. This will take time to reach - listen to your body and get there in your own pace. The ideal time to break your dry fast would be approximately 6pm to 7pm

And At Night Time...

Be sure to completely stop eating by 8pm (latest) so your body can prepare for a good night's sleep, rest and recovery.

DAY 14: DAILY TIP

"Ensure any amalgam fillings in your teeth are replaced with composite fillings – preferably by a holistic dentist. Metal poisoning is a common trigger for inner dysfunction and dis-ease."

DAY STRUCTURE REMINDERS

For The Morning...

Continuing your dry fast from your night sleep is a good idea. Work towards fasting up until at least 12pm. As your body adapts, start to increase this - the later you break your fast - the better.

In The Afternoon...

When you do finally decide to open your fast - focus on hydration. Spring water is a good start or slow-juiced fruits (e.g. berries, melons, citrus). Alternatively, eating soaked dates or your favourite fruits will suffice.

Evening Feast...

Work towards dry fasting for 23 hours and eating for 1 hour each day. This will take time to reach - listen to your body and get there in your own pace. The ideal time to break your dry fast would be approximately 6pm to 7pm

And At Night Time...

Be sure to completely stop eating by 8pm (latest) so your body can prepare for a good night's sleep, rest and recovery.

DAY 15: DAILY TIP

"Use parsley to detoxify mercury out of your body. Coupled with dry fasting, citrus fruits slow-juiced are also very good at pulling toxic waste out of your lymphatic system through your kidneys"

DAY STRUCTURE REMINDERS

For The Morning...

Continuing your dry fast from your night sleep is a good idea. Work towards fasting up until at least 12pm. As your body adapts, start to increase this - the later you break your fast - the better.

In The Afternoon...

When you do finally decide to open your fast - focus on hydration. Spring water is a good start or slow-juiced fruits (e.g. berries, melons, citrus). Alternatively, eating soaked dates or your favourite fruits will suffice.

Evening Feast...

Work towards dry fasting for 23 hours and eating for 1 hour each day. This will take time to reach - listen to your body and get there in your own pace. The ideal time to break your dry fast would be approximately 6pm to 7pm

And At Night Time...

Be sure to completely stop eating by 8pm (latest) so your body can prepare for a good night's sleep, rest and recovery.

DAY 16: DAILY TIP

"Sleep is very vital for your healing. Wind down by 7pm and aim to be in bed by 10pm to 10:30pm (if possible). During the initial stages of this protocol, you may sleep at points throughout the day as your body works on healing"

DAY STRUCTURE REMINDERS

For The Morning...

Continuing your dry fast from your night sleep is a good idea. Work towards fasting up until at least 12pm. As your body adapts, start to increase this - the later you break your fast - the better.

In The Afternoon...

When you do finally decide to open your fast - focus on hydration. Spring water is a good start or slow-juiced fruits (e.g. berries, melons, citrus). Alternatively, eating soaked dates or your favourite fruits will suffice.

Evening Feast...

Work towards dry fasting for 23 hours and eating for 1 hour each day. This will take time to reach - listen to your body and get there in your own pace. The ideal time to break your dry fast would be approximately 6pm to 7pm

And At Night Time...

Be sure to completely stop eating by 8pm (latest) so your body can prepare for a good night's sleep, rest and recovery.

DAY 17: DAILY TIP

"Keep a positive mindset - repeat positive affirmations daily. Remain persistent. Remind yourself that everything is possible & you WILL achieve your desired goals."

DAY STRUCTURE REMINDERS

For The Morning...

Continuing your dry fast from your night sleep is a good idea. Work towards fasting up until at least 12pm. As your body adapts, start to increase this - the later you break your fast - the better.

In The Afternoon...

When you do finally decide to open your fast - focus on hydration. Spring water is a good start or slow-juiced fruits (e.g. berries, melons, citrus). Alternatively, eating soaked dates or your favourite fruits will suffice.

Evening Feast...

Work towards dry fasting for 23 hours and eating for 1 hour each day. This will take time to reach - listen to your body and get there in your own pace. The ideal time to break your dry fast would be approximately 6pm to 7pm

And At Night Time...

Be sure to completely stop eating by 8pm (latest) so your body can prepare for a good night's sleep, rest and recovery.

DAY 18: DAILY TIP

"Get yourself an accountability partner to complete a 3 month detox with.
Start with 7 days and work your way up.
It will be fun and motivating completing it with somebody (or a group) ...or of course you can go it alone."

DAY STRUCTURE REMINDERS

For The Morning...

Continuing your dry fast from your night sleep is a good idea. Work towards fasting up until at least 12pm. As your body adapts, start to increase this - the later you break your fast - the better.

In The Afternoon...

When you do finally decide to open your fast - focus on hydration. Spring water is a good start or slow-juiced fruits (e.g. berries, melons, citrus). Alternatively, eating soaked dates or your favourite fruits will suffice.

Evening Feast...

Work towards dry fasting for 23 hours and eating for 1 hour each day. This will take time to reach - listen to your body and get there in your own pace. The ideal time to break your dry fast would be approximately 6pm to 7pm

And At Night Time...

Be sure to completely stop eating by 8pm (latest) so your body can prepare for a good night's sleep, rest and recovery.

DAY 19: DAILY TIP

"Remember when starting out, it is important to keep yourself hydrated throughout the day. Spring Water is a good start - and slow/cold pressed juice is also very powerful."

DAY STRUCTURE REMINDERS

For The Morning...

Continuing your dry fast from your night sleep is a good idea. Work towards fasting up until at least 12pm. As your body adapts, start to increase this - the later you break your fast - the better.

In The Afternoon...

When you do finally decide to open your fast - focus on hydration. Spring water is a good start or slow-juiced fruits (e.g. berries, melons, citrus). Alternatively, eating soaked dates or your favourite fruits will suffice.

Evening Feast...

Work towards dry fasting for 23 hours and eating for 1 hour each day. This will take time to reach - listen to your body and get there in your own pace. The ideal time to break your dry fast would be approximately 6pm to 7pm

And At Night Time...

Be sure to completely stop eating by 8pm (latest) so your body can prepare for a good night's sleep, rest and recovery.

DAY 20: DAILY TIP

"Eat melons/ watermelons separately, and before any other fruit as they digest faster and we want to limit fermentation (acidity) which can occur if other fruits are mixed in."

DAY STRUCTURE REMINDERS

For The Morning...

Continuing your dry fast from your night sleep is a good idea. Work towards fasting up until at least 12pm. As your body adapts, start to increase this - the later you break your fast - the better.

In The Afternoon...

When you do finally decide to open your fast - focus on hydration. Spring water is a good start or slow-juiced fruits (e.g. berries, melons, citrus). Alternatively, eating soaked dates or your favourite fruits will suffice.

Evening Feast...

Work towards dry fasting for 23 hours and eating for 1 hour each day. This will take time to reach - listen to your body and get there in your own pace. The ideal time to break your dry fast would be approximately 6pm to 7pm

And At Night Time...

Be sure to completely stop eating by 8pm (latest) so your body can prepare for a good night's sleep, rest and recovery.

DAY 21: DAILY TIP

"Stay focussed on the end goal of removing mucus & toxins from your body and feeling wonderful! Look forward to being full of vitality and dis-ease free once again"

DAY STRUCTURE REMINDERS

For The Morning...

Continuing your dry fast from your night sleep is a good idea. Work towards fasting up until at least 12pm. As your body adapts, start to increase this - the later you break your fast - the better.

In The Afternoon...

When you do finally decide to open your fast - focus on hydration. Spring water is a good start or slow-juiced fruits (e.g. berries, melons, citrus). Alternatively, eating soaked dates or your favourite fruits will suffice.

Evening Feast...

Work towards dry fasting for 23 hours and eating for 1 hour each day. This will take time to reach - listen to your body and get there in your own pace. The ideal time to break your dry fast would be approximately 6pm to 7pm

And At Night Time...

Be sure to completely stop eating by 8pm (latest) so your body can prepare for a good night's sleep, rest and recovery.

DAY 22: DAILY TIP

"Meditate and perform deep breathing exercises in order to help yourself remain present minded and on track. Perform these techniques throughout the day but also during any challenging times that you may come to face."

DAY STRUCTURE REMINDERS

For The Morning...

Continuing your dry fast from your night sleep is a good idea. Work towards fasting up until at least 12pm. As your body adapts, start to increase this - the later you break your fast - the better.

In The Afternoon...

When you do finally decide to open your fast - focus on hydration. Spring water is a good start or slow-juiced fruits (e.g. berries, melons, citrus). Alternatively, eating soaked dates or your favourite fruits will suffice.

Evening Feast...

Work towards dry fasting for 23 hours and eating for 1 hour each day. This will take time to reach - listen to your body and get there in your own pace. The ideal time to break your dry fast would be approximately 6pm to 7pm

And At Night Time...

Be sure to completely stop eating by 8pm (latest) so your body can prepare for a good night's sleep, rest and recovery.

DAY 23: DAILY TIP

"Join a few like-minded communities – there are many juicing and raw vegan based groups, both online and offline. Being part of a community can help motivate you to reach your goals. You will also learn a great amount from others. Seeing others succeed is empowering."

DAY STRUCTURE REMINDERS

For The Morning...

Continuing your dry fast from your night sleep is a good idea. Work towards fasting up until at least 12pm. As your body adapts, start to increase this - the later you break your fast - the better.

In The Afternoon...

When you do finally decide to open your fast - focus on hydration. Spring water is a good start or slow-juiced fruits (e.g. berries, melons, citrus). Alternatively, eating soaked dates or your favourite fruits will suffice.

Evening Feast...

Work towards dry fasting for 23 hours and eating for 1 hour each day. This will take time to reach - listen to your body and get there in your own pace. The ideal time to break your dry fast would be approximately 6pm to 7pm

And At Night Time...

Be sure to completely stop eating by 8pm (latest) so your body can prepare for a good night's sleep, rest and recovery.

DAY 24: DAILY TIP

"If you are struggling to cope with hunger pangs in the early stages, try some dates or dried apricots, prunes, or raisins, with a cup of herbal tea. However, these pangs will disappear once your body adjusts to your new routine."

DAY STRUCTURE REMINDERS

For The Morning...

Continuing your dry fast from your night sleep is a good idea. Work towards fasting up until at least 12pm. As your body adapts, start to increase this - the later you break your fast - the better.

In The Afternoon...

When you do finally decide to open your fast - focus on hydration. Spring water is a good start or slow-juiced fruits (e.g. berries, melons, citrus). Alternatively, eating soaked dates or your favourite fruits will suffice.

Evening Feast...

Work towards dry fasting for 23 hours and eating for 1 hour each day. This will take time to reach - listen to your body and get there in your own pace. The ideal time to break your dry fast would be approximately 6pm to 7pm

And At Night Time...

Be sure to completely stop eating by 8pm (latest) so your body can prepare for a good night's sleep, rest and recovery.

DAY 25: DAILY TIP

"Get into a routine of regularly buying fresh fruit (or grow your own if weather permits) to keep your supplies up. Local wholesale markets do also clear fruit on Fridays (if they are closed for the weekend) at a lower price, so they are worth a visit."

DAY STRUCTURE REMINDERS

For The Morning...

Continuing your dry fast from your night sleep is a good idea. Work towards fasting up until at least 12pm. As your body adapts, start to increase this - the later you break your fast - the better.

In The Afternoon...

When you do finally decide to open your fast - focus on hydration. Spring water is a good start or slow-juiced fruits (e.g. berries, melons, citrus). Alternatively, eating soaked dates or your favourite fruits will suffice.

Evening Feast...

Work towards dry fasting for 23 hours and eating for 1 hour each day. This will take time to reach - listen to your body and get there in your own pace. The ideal time to break your dry fast would be approximately 6pm to 7pm

And At Night Time...

Be sure to completely stop eating by 8pm (latest) so your body can prepare for a good night's sleep, rest and recovery.

DAY 26: DAILY TIP

"Regularly remind yourself about the great rewards and benefits that you will experience by keeping up this detoxification process. Imagine the lives you could save as a result of healing yourself."

DAY STRUCTURE REMINDERS

For The Morning...

Continuing your dry fast from your night sleep is a good idea. Work towards fasting up until at least 12pm. As your body adapts, start to increase this - the later you break your fast - the better.

In The Afternoon...

When you do finally decide to open your fast - focus on hydration. Spring water is a good start or slow-juiced fruits (e.g. berries, melons, citrus). Alternatively, eating soaked dates or your favourite fruits will suffice.

Evening Feast...

Work towards dry fasting for 23 hours and eating for 1 hour each day. This will take time to reach - listen to your body and get there in your own pace. The ideal time to break your dry fast would be approximately 6pm to 7pm

And At Night Time...

Be sure to completely stop eating by 8pm (latest) so your body can prepare for a good night's sleep, rest and recovery.

DAY 27: DAILY TIP

"Keep your teeth brushed and flossed regularly – at least twice a day (morning & night) to keep them healthy for your fruit sessions. You will notice an improvement in your dental health with this raw/fruit diet."

DAY STRUCTURE REMINDERS

For The Morning...

Continuing your dry fast from your night sleep is a good idea. Work towards fasting up until at least 12pm. As your body adapts, start to increase this - the later you break your fast - the better.

In The Afternoon...

When you do finally decide to open your fast - focus on hydration. Spring water is a good start or slow-juiced fruits (e.g. berries, melons, citrus). Alternatively, eating soaked dates or your favourite fruits will suffice.

Evening Feast...

Work towards dry fasting for 23 hours and eating for 1 hour each day. This will take time to reach - listen to your body and get there in your own pace. The ideal time to break your dry fast would be approximately 6pm to 7pm

And At Night Time...

Be sure to completely stop eating by 8pm (latest) so your body can prepare for a good night's sleep, rest and recovery.

DAY 28: DAILY TIP

"Be motivated by the vision of becoming an example for others to learn from and follow. You could change the lives of family and friends by showing them your own improvements."

DAY STRUCTURE REMINDERS

For The Morning...

Continuing your dry fast from your night sleep is a good idea. Work towards fasting up until at least 12pm. As your body adapts, start to increase this - the later you break your fast - the better.

In The Afternoon...

When you do finally decide to open your fast - focus on hydration. Spring water is a good start or slow-juiced fruits (e.g. berries, melons, citrus). Alternatively, eating soaked dates or your favourite fruits will suffice.

Evening Feast...

Work towards dry fasting for 23 hours and eating for 1 hour each day. This will take time to reach - listen to your body and get there in your own pace. The ideal time to break your dry fast would be approximately 6pm to 7pm

And At Night Time...

Be sure to completely stop eating by 8pm (latest) so your body can prepare for a good night's sleep, rest and recovery.

DAY 29: DAILY TIP

"Embrace your achievements and wonderful results – feel and appreciate the difference within you as a result of this new routine. Notice how your personal agility and fitness has improved. Feel the improved energy levels."

DAY STRUCTURE REMINDERS

For The Morning...

Continuing your dry fast from your night sleep is a good idea. Work towards fasting up until at least 12pm. As your body adapts, start to increase this - the later you break your fast - the better.

In The Afternoon...

When you do finally decide to open your fast - focus on hydration. Spring water is a good start or slow-juiced fruits (e.g. berries, melons, citrus). Alternatively, eating soaked dates or your favourite fruits will suffice.

Evening Feast...

Work towards dry fasting for 23 hours and eating for 1 hour each day. This will take time to reach - listen to your body and get there in your own pace. The ideal time to break your dry fast would be approximately 6pm to 7pm

And At Night Time...

Be sure to completely stop eating by 8pm (latest) so your body can prepare for a good night's sleep, rest and recovery.

DAY 30: DAILY TIP

"Buy fruit in bulk where possible so you have ample supplies for a week or two in advance. If in a hot climate, you could even freeze your fruit or make ice lollies out of it (crush & freeze). Immerse yourself in fruit so it becomes your only option."

CPSIA information can be obtained
at www.ICGtesting.com
Printed in the USA
BVHW041629130919
558402BV00008B/1527/P

9 781395 40458